Introduction

Sugar has become an integral part of our modern diet, found in a wide array of foods and beverages. While our bodies require small amounts of sugar for energy, excessive consumption of added sugars has been linked to a range of chronic diseases that pose significant health risks. Understanding the connection between sugar and chronic diseases is crucial for promoting better health and making informed dietary choices.

In this introductory book, we will delve into the relationship between sugar and chronic diseases, exploring the scientific evidence and shedding light on the impact of excessive sugar consumption on our well-being. Through a comprehensive exploration of various chronic conditions, we will uncover the role of sugar as a contributing factor and discuss strategies to mitigate its detrimental effects.

Chapter 1: The Sweet Temptation

- Understanding different types of sugars and their sources
- The prevalence of added sugars in our food supply
- How excessive sugar consumption has become a global health concern

Chapter 2: The Bitter Consequences: Obesity and Metabolic Syndrome

- The role of sugar in the development of obesity
- The link between sugar and metabolic syndrome
- Exploring insulin resistance and its connection to chronic diseases

Chapter 3: Sweet Tooth and Diabetes

- The impact of sugar on blood sugar levels and insulin production
- Sugar consumption as a risk factor for type 2 diabetes

- Strategies for preventing and managing diabetes through sugar control

Chapter 4: The Sour Truth: Cardiovascular Diseases

- The influence of sugar on heart health and blood lipid profiles
- Understanding the relationship between sugar and hypertension
- The role of sugar in promoting inflammation and oxidative stress

Chapter 5: Sugar and the Silent Threat: Non-Alcoholic Fatty Liver Disease

- The connection between excessive sugar intake and liver fat accumulation
- Understanding the progression from fatty liver to more severe liver conditions
- Strategies for reducing sugar consumption to protect liver health

Chapter 6: Sugar's Impact on Mental Health and Cognitive Function

- Exploring the link between sugar and mental health conditions like depression and anxiety
- The effect of sugar on cognitive function, memory, and brain health
- Promoting emotional well-being and mental clarity through sugar management

Chapter 7: Breaking Free from the Sugar Trap: Strategies for a Healthier Life

- Practical tips for reducing sugar intake and making healthier dietary choices
- Navigating food labels and identifying hidden sugars in processed foods
- Embracing a balanced and sustainable approach to sugar consumption

Conclusion: A Sweet and Balanced Future

- The importance of awareness and education in combating the sugar-related chronic disease epidemic
- Empowering individuals to take control of their health through informed choices
- Promoting a society that prioritizes health and well-being by addressing excessive sugar consumption

Chapter 1: The Sweet Temptation

What Is Processed Sugar?

Processed sugar refers to sugars that have undergone significant refining and processing to extract them from their natural sources. It typically refers to granulated sugar, which is the most commonly used form of sugar in households and the food industry. Here are some common types of processed sugars:

- **Granulated sugar:** This is the white or brown sugar found in most households. It is made from either sugarcane or sugar beets. The juice extracted from the plants undergoes multiple refining processes to remove impurities and moisture, resulting in refined white or brown sugar.

- **Powdered sugar:** Also known as confectioner's sugar or icing sugar, it is a finely ground form of sugar that is often used for dusting or making icing. It is made by pulverizing granulated sugar and adding a small amount of cornstarch to prevent clumping.

- **High-fructose corn syrup (HFCS):** HFCS is a liquid sweetener derived from corn starch. It undergoes enzymatic processes to convert the glucose in corn syrup into fructose, resulting in a syrup that is sweeter than regular sugar. It is commonly used in processed foods and beverages.

- ***Corn syrup:*** Corn syrup is a thick, sticky syrup made from cornstarch. It is primarily composed of glucose and is used as a sweetener in various processed foods and candies.

- ***Molasses:*** Molasses is a byproduct of the sugar refining process. It is thick, dark, and has a distinct flavor. Molasses is often used in baking, marinades, and some traditional desserts.

Processed sugars are often added to a wide range of processed and packaged foods, including soft drinks, desserts, pastries, candies, sauces, and condiments. These added sugars contribute to the sweet taste of these foods but provide little to no nutritional value.

It's important to read food labels and be aware of the various names and forms of processed sugars to make informed choices about your sugar consumption.

Artificial Sweeteners

Artificial sweeteners are synthetic sugar substitutes that provide sweetness without the calories or impact on blood sugar levels associated with regular sugar. They are commonly used as alternatives to sugar in various food and beverage products. Here are some common types of artificial sweeteners:

Aspartame: Aspartame is one of the most widely used artificial sweeteners. It is found in many sugar-free or "diet" products, including soft drinks, chewing gum, and desserts. Aspartame is composed of two amino acids and is about 200 times sweeter than sugar.

Sucralose: Sucralose is another popular artificial sweetener. It is derived from sugar and is approximately 600 times sweeter than sugar. Sucralose is heat-stable and can be used in a variety of foods and beverages, including baked goods and beverages.

Saccharin: Saccharin has been used as an artificial sweetener for many years. It is intensely sweet and has a bitter aftertaste. Saccharin is often found in diet sodas, tabletop sweeteners, and other processed foods.

Acesulfame Potassium (Ace-K): Acesulfame potassium is a calorie-free sweetener that is approximately 200 times sweeter than sugar. It is often used in combination with other artificial sweeteners to enhance sweetness in food and beverage products.

Neotame: Neotame is a highly potent artificial sweetener that is approximately 7,000 to 13,000 times sweeter than sugar. It is used in small amounts and is found in various processed foods and beverages.

Processed foods

Processed foods often contain added sugars as a common ingredient. These added sugars are used to enhance flavor, extend shelf life, and improve the texture of processed food products. Here are some examples of processed foods that commonly contain added sugars:

Soft Drinks and Fruit Juices: Sugary soft drinks and fruit juices are notorious for their high sugar content. They can contribute to excessive sugar intake and have been linked to various health issues such as obesity, type 2 diabetes, and tooth decay.

Breakfast Cereals: Many breakfast cereals, especially those marketed towards children, contain significant amounts of added sugars. It's important to check the nutrition labels and choose cereals with lower sugar content or opt for healthier alternatives like whole grain cereals or oatmeal.

Baked Goods: Cookies, cakes, pastries, and other baked goods often contain added sugars to enhance sweetness and improve texture. These treats can be high in calories and should be consumed in moderation.

Snack Bars and Granola Bars: Snack bars and granola bars can be convenient on-the-go options, but they can also be high in added sugars. Reading the nutrition labels and choosing bars with less added sugars or opting for homemade versions with natural sweeteners can be healthier alternatives.

Sauces, Dressings, and Condiments: Many sauces, dressings, and condiments, such as ketchup, barbecue sauce, and salad dressings, contain added sugars. These hidden sources of sugar can contribute to daily sugar intake. Opt for homemade or low-sugar versions when possible.

Sweetened Yogurt and Dairy Products: Flavored yogurts, flavored milk, and other sweetened dairy products often contain added sugars. Choosing plain or unsweetened versions and adding fresh fruits or natural sweeteners like honey or stevia can help reduce sugar intake.

Ready-to-Eat Meals and Processed Meats: Ready-to-eat meals, processed meats like sausages and deli meats, and certain sauces used in these products can contain added sugars. Reading labels and selecting options with lower sugar content or preparing homemade meals with fresh ingredients can be healthier choices.

Alternative to Processed Sugar

If you're looking for alternatives to processed sugar, there are several natural sweeteners that you can consider. These alternatives can provide sweetness to your dishes while offering some potential benefits over refined sugar. Here are some popular alternatives:

Honey: Honey is a natural sweetener produced by bees. It contains small amounts of vitamins, minerals, and antioxidants. However, it is still high in sugar and should be used in moderation.

Sugar cane juice

Is a popular and refreshing beverage made from the extract of freshly squeezed sugar cane stalks. It is commonly consumed in many parts of the world, including Kenya. Here are some key points about sugar cane juice:

Natural Sweetness: Sugar cane juice has a naturally sweet taste due to the high sugar content present in sugar cane stalks. It provides a refreshing burst of sweetness, similar to other fruit juices.

Hydration: Sugar cane juice is a hydrating beverage as it primarily consists of water. It can help quench thirst and replenish fluids in hot weather or after physical activity.

Nutrient Content: Sugar cane juice contains essential nutrients such as carbohydrates, calcium, magnesium, potassium, and iron. However, the exact nutrient composition can vary based on factors like the variety of sugarcane and the extraction process.

Antioxidants: Sugar cane juice contains antioxidants, including flavonoids and phenolic compounds, which have potential health benefits. These antioxidants help in combating oxidative stress and reducing the risk of certain diseases.

Natural Energy Boost: Due to its high sugar content, sugar cane juice can provide a quick source of natural energy. However, it is important to consume it in moderation, especially for individuals with diabetes or those watching their sugar intake.

Freshly Squeezed Preferred: It is recommended to consume sugar cane juice when it is freshly extracted to retain its freshness and nutritional value. Some vendors may add lime juice or other flavors to enhance the taste.

Maple Syrup: Maple syrup is derived from the sap of maple trees. It has a distinct flavor and contains some minerals like manganese and zinc. Choose 100% pure maple syrup without any added sugars or artificial ingredients.

Stevia: Stevia is a plant-based sweetener extracted from the leaves of the Stevia rebaudiana plant. It is intensely sweet but has zero calories. Look for pure stevia extract or stevia-based sweeteners without added fillers or additives.

Coconut Sugar: Coconut sugar is made from the sap of coconut palm trees. It retains some nutrients found in the coconut palm, including potassium, iron, and zinc. However, it is still a sugar and should be used in moderation.

Date Sugar: Date sugar is made from dried and ground dates. It retains the fiber and nutrients present in dates, making it a more wholesome alternative. However, it does not dissolve well and may not be suitable for all recipes.

Monk Fruit Sweetener: Monk fruit sweetener is derived from the monk fruit and is known for its intense sweetness. It has zero calories and does not raise blood sugar levels. Look for pure monk fruit extract or blends without added sugars or additives.

Chapter 2: The Bitter Consequences: Obesity and Metabolic Syndrome.

Obesity and metabolic syndrome are two interconnected health conditions that have reached epidemic proportions worldwide. Excessive sugar consumption is recognized as a significant contributing factor to the development of both obesity and metabolic syndrome. Let's explore the bitter consequences of these conditions:

Obesity:

Excessive sugar consumption, particularly in the form of added sugars and sugary beverages, has been closely linked to weight gain and obesity. Here's how sugar contributes to obesity:

a. High-Calorie Content: Sugary foods and drinks are typically high in calories but offer little nutritional value. Consuming them in excess leads to an imbalance between calorie intake and expenditure, resulting in weight gain.

b. Increased Appetite and Overeating: Consuming sugary foods triggers a rapid rise in blood sugar levels, followed by a sharp drop. This fluctuation can lead to increased hunger and cravings, causing individuals to consume more calories than needed.

c. Insulin Resistance: Frequent consumption of high-sugar foods can lead to insulin resistance, where the body's cells become less responsive to the hormone insulin. Insulin resistance interferes with the body's ability to regulate blood sugar levels and can promote fat storage, particularly in the abdominal area.

Metabolic Syndrome:

Metabolic syndrome is a cluster of health conditions that often occur together and significantly increase the risk of cardiovascular disease, type 2 diabetes, and other chronic illnesses. Excessive sugar consumption contributes to the development of metabolic syndrome through various mechanisms:

a. Insulin Resistance: As mentioned earlier, excessive sugar consumption can lead to insulin resistance. Insulin resistance is a key component of metabolic syndrome, contributing to elevated blood sugar levels, abnormal blood lipid profiles, and increased cardiovascular risk.

b. Abdominal Obesity: Excessive sugar intake can promote weight gain, particularly around the abdominal area. This visceral fat accumulation is associated with metabolic disturbances, including insulin resistance, high blood pressure, and dyslipidemia - all hallmark features of metabolic syndrome.

c. Elevated Blood Pressure: A high-sugar diet has been linked to increased blood pressure levels, which is a crucial criterion for diagnosing metabolic syndrome. The combination of insulin resistance, excess weight, and the impact of sugar on blood vessel function can contribute to elevated blood pressure.

d. Dyslipidemia: Excessive sugar consumption, especially in the form of fructose, can raise triglyceride levels and reduce high-density lipoprotein (HDL) cholesterol levels. This lipid profile imbalance contributes to dyslipidemia, another characteristic feature of metabolic syndrome.

The bitter consequences of obesity and metabolic syndrome extend far beyond physical appearance. These conditions significantly increase the risk of chronic diseases, such as type 2 diabetes, cardiovascular disease, stroke, and certain cancers. Understanding the role of excessive sugar consumption in the development of obesity and metabolic syndrome is essential for implementing preventive measures and adopting healthier dietary patterns.

By reducing sugar intake, adopting a balanced diet rich in whole foods, and incorporating regular physical activity, individuals can mitigate the risks of obesity and metabolic syndrome, promoting better overall health and well-being

Chapter 3: Sweet Tooth and Diabetes

The prevalence of diabetes has reached epidemic proportions worldwide, with millions of individuals affected by this chronic metabolic disorder. While genetics and lifestyle factors play a role in diabetes development, the impact of excessive sugar consumption, particularly in individuals with a "sweet tooth," cannot be ignored.

Weight gain and obesity.

Added sugar is high in calories but low in nutrients, so consuming too much can lead to weight gain and obesity. Obesity is a major risk factor for many chronic diseases, including heart disease, type 2 diabetes, and some types of cancer.

Scientific research has established a clear link between the consumption of processed sugar and weight gain/obesity. Here's some evidence supporting this connection:

1. ***Caloric Density:*** Processed sugar is highly caloric and offers little to no nutritional value. Consuming foods and beverages high in added sugars can lead to an excessive calorie intake, which can contribute to weight gain over time.

2. ***Increased Appetite and Overeating:*** High sugar intake can disrupt appetite regulation mechanisms in the body, leading to increased hunger and a higher likelihood of overeating.

Sugar-rich foods are often less filling and can result in a higher overall caloric intake.

3. ***Effects on Hormones:*** Consumption of processed sugar, particularly fructose, can affect hormone regulation related to appetite control and fat storage. It can lead to insulin resistance, impaired leptin signaling (the hormone responsible for satiety), and increased production of the hunger hormone ghrelin.

4. ***Sugar-Sweetened Beverages:*** Regular consumption of sugar-sweetened beverages, such as soda and fruit juices, has been strongly linked to weight gain and obesity. These beverages provide a significant amount of added sugars and calories, contributing to an increased risk of excessive weight gain.

5. ***Body Fat Accumulation:*** Excess consumption of processed sugar, especially in the form of fructose, can contribute to increased fat deposition, particularly visceral fat (fat around the abdominal organs). Visceral fat is associated with a higher risk of metabolic disorders and obesity-related health complications.

These studies and others provide strong evidence that excessive consumption of processed sugar, especially in the form of added sugars and sugar-sweetened beverages, can contribute to weight gain and obesity. Reducing the intake of processed sugar is an important step in managing weight and promoting overall health.

Type 2 diabetes.

High intake of added sugar has been linked to an increased risk of type 2 diabetes. This is because processed sugar can lead to spikes in blood sugar levels, which can damage cells in the pancreas and make it difficult for the body to produce insulin. Insulin is a hormone that helps the body use glucose for energy.

While processed sugar is not the sole cause of type 2 diabetes, there is evidence to suggest that excessive consumption of processed sugar, especially in the form of added sugars, can increase the risk of developing the condition. Here's some information supporting this connection:

1. ***Insulin Resistance:*** High sugar intake, particularly from sources with a high glycemic index, can contribute to insulin resistance. Insulin resistance is a condition in which cells become less responsive to the effects of insulin, leading to elevated blood sugar levels and an increased risk of developing type 2 diabetes.

2. ***Increased Risk of Obesity:*** High sugar consumption is associated with weight gain and obesity, which are significant risk factors for the development of type 2 diabetes. Excess body weight, especially abdominal obesity, can impair insulin sensitivity and increase the likelihood of developing insulin resistance.

3. ***Beta Cell Dysfunction:*** Beta cells in the pancreas are responsible for producing and secreting insulin. Chronic high sugar intake may contribute to the dysfunction and decreased viability of beta cells, impairing insulin production and secretion, thereby increasing the risk of developing type 2 diabetes.

4. ***Impaired Glucose Tolerance:*** Regular consumption of high-sugar foods and beverages can lead to elevated blood sugar levels, potentially leading to impaired glucose tolerance. Prolonged periods of elevated blood sugar levels can contribute to the development of insulin resistance and type 2 diabetes.

It's important to note that while processed sugar can contribute to the risk of developing type 2 diabetes, other factors such as genetic predisposition, sedentary lifestyle, and overall dietary patterns also play significant roles. A balanced diet, regular physical activity, and maintaining a healthy weight are crucial for reducing the risk of type 2 diabetes. If you have concerns about your sugar consumption or risk of diabetes, it's recommended to consult with a healthcare professional for personalized advice.

Chapter 4: The Sour Truth: Cardiovascular Diseases

Cardiovascular diseases (CVD) remain the leading cause of mortality globally, contributing to millions of deaths each year. While multiple factors contribute to the development of CVD, emerging research has shed light on the detrimental impact of excessive sugar consumption on cardiovascular health.

Heart disease.

Consuming too much added sugar can raise blood pressure, cholesterol levels, and inflammation. These factors can all increase the risk of heart disease.

Processed sugar can contribute to heart disease in a number of ways.

1. ***High blood pressure.*** Consuming too much processed sugar can lead to high blood pressure, a major risk factor for heart disease. This is because sugar can cause the body to retain fluids, which can put extra strain on the heart.

2. ***High cholesterol levels.*** Eating too much processed sugar can also lead to high cholesterol levels, another risk factor for heart disease. This is because sugar can increase the

production of triglycerides, a type of fat that can build up in the arteries and narrow them.

3. **Inflammation.** Consuming too much processed sugar can also lead to inflammation, which can damage the lining of the arteries and make them more likely to develop plaque. Plaque is a fatty buildup that can narrow the arteries and increase the risk of heart attack or stroke.

4. **Weight gain and obesity.** Weight gain and obesity are major risk factors for heart disease. Consuming too much processed sugar can lead to weight gain and obesity because it is high in calories and low in nutrients.

5. **Type 2 diabetes.** Type 2 diabetes is another major risk factor for heart disease. Consuming too much processed sugar can increase the risk of type 2 diabetes because it can lead to insulin resistance. Insulin is a hormone that helps the body use glucose for energy. When cells become resistant to insulin, glucose builds up in the bloodstream, which can lead to type 2 diabetes.

Stroke.

Stroke is a leading cause of death worldwide. High intake of added sugar has been linked to an increased risk of stroke, especially in women.Processed sugar can increase the risk of stroke in a few ways.

1. **High blood pressure.** Consuming too much processed sugar can lead to high blood pressure, which is a major risk factor for stroke. This is because sugar can cause the body to retain fluids, which can put extra strain on the heart. High blood pressure can damage the blood vessels in the brain, making them more likely to rupture or clot.

2. ***High cholesterol levels.*** Eating too much processed sugar can also lead to high cholesterol levels, another risk factor for stroke. This is because sugar can increase the production of triglycerides, a type of fat that can build up in the arteries and narrow them. Narrowed arteries make it harder for blood to flow to the brain, which can increase the risk of stroke.

3. ***Inflammation.*** Consuming too much processed sugar can also lead to inflammation, which can damage the lining of the arteries and make them more likely to develop plaque. Plaque is a fatty buildup that can narrow the arteries and increase the risk of stroke.

4. ***Weight gain and obesity.*** Weight gain and obesity are major risk factors for stroke. Consuming too much processed sugar can lead to weight gain and obesity because it is high in calories and low in nutrients. Obesity can increase the risk of stroke by increasing the risk of high blood pressure, high cholesterol levels, and inflammation.

5. ***Type 2 diabetes.*** Type 2 diabetes is another major risk factor for stroke. Consuming too much processed sugar can increase the risk of type 2 diabetes because it can lead to insulin resistance. Insulin is a hormone that helps the body use glucose for energy. When cells become resistant to insulin, glucose builds up in the bloodstream, which can increase the risk of stroke.

6. ***Obesity:*** Consuming large amounts of sugar can contribute to weight gain and obesity. Obesity is a significant risk factor for cardiovascular diseases such as heart disease and stroke.

7. ***Insulin resistance and diabetes:*** Consuming excessive amounts of sugar can lead to insulin resistance, where the body becomes less responsive to insulin. Insulin resistance is a precursor to type 2 diabetes, which is associated with an increased risk of cardiovascular diseases.

8. ***Inflammation:*** A diet high in sugar can trigger inflammation in the body. Chronic inflammation plays a role in the development of atherosclerosis (hardening of the arteries) and can increase the risk of heart disease.

9. ***Dyslipidemia:*** Excessive sugar intake, particularly in the form of fructose, can contribute to dyslipidemia, which is an abnormal lipid profile characterized by increased levels of triglycerides and decreased levels of HDL (good) cholesterol. Dyslipidemia is a risk factor for cardiovascular diseases.

It's important to note that cardiovascular diseases are complex conditions influenced by multiple factors, including genetics, lifestyle choices, and overall diet quality. While processed sugar is a contributing factor, it is just one piece of the puzzle. Maintaining a balanced diet low in added sugars, along with regular exercise, managing weight, and adopting a heart-healthy lifestyle, can help reduce the risk of cardiovascular diseases.

Chapter 5: Sugar and the Silent Threat: Non-Alcoholic Fatty Liver Disease

Non-Alcoholic Fatty Liver Disease (NAFLD) is a prevalent and often silent condition characterized by the accumulation of fat in the liver, unrelated to excessive alcohol consumption. Emerging research suggests that excessive sugar consumption plays a significant role in the development and progression of NAFLD.

Non-alcoholic fatty liver disease (NAFLD). NAFLD is a condition in which fat builds up in the liver. It is a major risk factor for liver disease, heart disease, and type 2 diabetes. High intake of added sugar has been linked to an increased risk of NAFLD.There is evidence to suggest that excessive consumption of processed sugar, particularly in the form of fructose, can contribute to the development of non-alcoholic fatty liver disease (NAFLD). Here's some information supporting this connection:

1. ***Increased Fat Accumulation:*** Consuming high amounts of sugar, especially fructose, can lead to the accumulation of fat in the liver. Excess fructose consumption promotes de novo lipogenesis, a process where the liver converts sugar into fat, contributing to the development of fatty liver.

2. ***Insulin Resistance and Metabolic Syndrome:*** Excessive sugar intake can lead to insulin resistance, impairing the ability of cells to respond to insulin properly. Insulin resistance is closely linked to the development of NAFLD and metabolic syndrome, a cluster of conditions that increase the risk of heart disease, type 2 diabetes, and liver disease.

3. ***Increased Inflammation and Oxidative Stress:*** High sugar consumption can promote inflammation and oxidative

stress in the liver, contributing to the progression of NAFLD. These processes can damage liver cells and exacerbate liver injury.

4. ***Altered Gut Microbiota:*** Excessive sugar intake can disrupt the balance of gut bacteria, leading to dysbiosis. Changes in gut microbiota composition and function have been associated with the development and progression of NAFLD.

It's important to note that NAFLD is a complex condition influenced by multiple factors, including genetics, overall diet, sedentary lifestyle, and other metabolic disorders. While excessive consumption of processed sugar can contribute to the development of NAFLD, it is essential to consider a comprehensive approach to liver health, including a balanced diet, regular physical activity, weight management, and overall healthy lifestyle choices.

Chapter 6: Mental Health and Cognitive Function

Depression.

Some studies have shown that high intake of added sugar may be linked to an increased risk of depression.While diet and nutrition can have an impact on mental health, it is important to note that depression is a complex condition with multifactorial causes. While excessive consumption of processed sugar may contribute to certain health issues, there is no direct causal relationship between processed sugar and depression.However, there are some indirect ways in which a diet high in processed sugar can potentially affect mental health:

__Blood sugar fluctuations:__ Consuming large amounts of processed sugar can cause rapid spikes and drops in blood sugar levels. These fluctuations can lead to feelings of fatigue, irritability, and mood swings, which may exacerbate symptoms of depression or increase the risk of developing depressive symptoms.

__Nutrient deficiencies:__ Diets high in processed sugar tend to be low in essential nutrients such as vitamins, minerals, and omega-3 fatty acids, which are important for brain health and the production of neurotransmitters involved in mood regulation. Inadequate intake of these nutrients can potentially impact mental well-being.

Chapter 7: Cancer

While some studies have suggested potential associations between high sugar intake and certain types of cancer, the overall evidence is limited and inconclusive.

However, it is widely accepted that a diet high in added sugars can contribute to weight gain and obesity. Obesity, in turn, is associated with an increased risk of developing certain types of cancer, including **breast, colorectal, endometrial, kidney, pancreatic, and liver cancers**. This association is more likely due to the overall impact of excess body weight and its effects on hormonal balance, chronic inflammation, and insulin resistance, rather than the direct effect of sugar consumption itself.

To reduce the risk of cancer and promote overall health, it is recommended to follow a balanced diet that includes a variety of whole foods, such as fruits, vegetables, whole grains, lean proteins, and healthy fats, while minimizing the intake of added sugars and processed foods. It is always advisable to consult with healthcare professionals or registered dietitians for personalized advice on nutrition and lifestyle choices to support cancer prevention and overall well-being.

Chapter 8: Dental issues

Processed sugars promote the growth of harmful bacteria in the mouth, leading to tooth decay and cavities. Regular consumption of sugary foods and drinks can increase the risk of dental problems and oral health issues.

Consuming excessive amounts of processed sugar can contribute to various dental issues. Here are some dental problems associated with high sugar intake:

Tooth Decay: The most common dental issue caused by sugar is tooth decay, also known as dental caries or cavities. Bacteria in the mouth feed on sugars and produce acids that erode tooth enamel, leading to decay. Over time, this can result in cavities and toothaches.

Enamel Erosion: Sugar-laden foods and beverages are often acidic as well. Acidic substances, combined with sugar, can lead to enamel erosion. Enamel is the protective outer layer of the teeth, and its erosion can make the teeth more sensitive and prone to damage.

Gum Disease: High sugar consumption can contribute to the development of gum disease, also known as periodontal disease. The bacteria in plaque, which forms on the teeth, thrive on sugar. Over time, this can lead to inflammation, gum recession, and even tooth loss if left untreated.

Bad Breath: Bacteria in the mouth thrive on sugar and release foul-smelling gases as a byproduct of their metabolic processes. Consequently, consuming excessive sugar can contribute to bad breath, or halitosis.

Discoloration: Dark-colored sugary beverages like cola and fruit juices can stain the teeth over time. These pigments, known as chromogens, can lead to surface stains and discoloration, impacting the appearance of your smile.

What Next?

It's important to note that not all sugars are created equal. Naturally occurring sugars found in fruits, vegetables, and dairy products come with fiber, vitamins, and minerals, which moderate their impact on blood sugar levels and offer some nutritional benefits.

To reduce the health risks associated with processed sugar consumption, it is advisable to limit the intake of sugary processed foods and beverages, read food labels to identify hidden sugars, and focus on a balanced diet that emphasizes whole foods, including fruits, vegetables, lean proteins, whole grains, and healthy fats. Moderation and mindful consumption of sugar can contribute to better overall health and well-being.

Chapter 9: Breaking Free from the Sugar Trap: Strategies for a Healthier Life

From weight gain and increased risk of chronic diseases to energy crashes and mood swings, the consequences of excessive sugar consumption are alarming.

Healthy Gut

A healthy gut plays a crucial role in our overall well-being. It is responsible for the digestion and absorption of nutrients, the synthesis of vitamins, and the support of a strong immune system. Here are some key factors and practices that contribute to a healthy gut:

Balanced Diet: Consuming a diverse and balanced diet is essential for a healthy gut. Include a variety of fruits, vegetables, whole grains, lean proteins, and healthy fats in your meals. This promotes the growth of beneficial gut bacteria and ensures a wide range of nutrients for optimal gut function.

Fiber-Rich Foods: Adequate fiber intake is crucial for maintaining a healthy gut. Fiber promotes regular bowel movements, helps prevent constipation, and supports the growth of beneficial gut bacteria. Include foods such as fruits, vegetables, whole grains, legumes, and nuts in your diet to boost your fiber intake.

Probiotics: Probiotics are beneficial bacteria that support a healthy gut. They can be found in fermented foods like yogurt, kefir, sauerkraut, and kimchi. Consuming these probiotic-rich foods helps restore and maintain a healthy balance of gut bacteria.

Prebiotics: Prebiotics are non-digestible fibers that act as food for beneficial gut bacteria. They help promote the growth and activity of these bacteria. Foods rich in prebiotics include garlic, onions, leeks, asparagus, bananas, and whole grains.

Hydration: Drinking an adequate amount of water is essential for maintaining a healthy gut. Water helps soften stool, supports digestion, and aids in the absorption of nutrients.

Minimize Stress: Chronic stress can disrupt the balance of bacteria in the gut and affect gut function. Engage in stress-reducing activities such as exercise, meditation, deep breathing, and adequate sleep to promote a healthy gut.

Limit Processed Foods and Added Sugars: Processed foods and added sugars can negatively impact the gut by promoting the growth of harmful bacteria. Minimize the intake of these foods and opt for whole, unprocessed foods instead.
Regular Physical Activity: Engaging in regular physical activity not only benefits overall health but also promotes a healthy gut. Exercise helps stimulate regular bowel movements, improves gut motility, and enhances gut microbial diversity.

Adequate Sleep: Prioritize getting enough sleep as it plays a vital role in maintaining a healthy gut. Poor sleep patterns have been linked to an imbalance in gut bacteria and increased risk of digestive issues.

Avoid Antibiotic Overuse: While antibiotics are necessary in certain situations, overuse can disrupt the balance of gut bacteria. Use antibiotics judiciously and follow healthcare professional's instructions when prescribed.

No Sugar Diet / Sugar Detox

A no sugar diet, also known as a sugar-free diet or sugar detox, is a dietary approach that involves avoiding or significantly reducing the consumption of added sugars and foods high in sugar content. This type of diet aims to minimize the intake of refined sugars and promote a healthier lifestyle. However, it's important to note that some natural sugars, such as those found in fruits and vegetables, are generally considered acceptable in moderation due to their accompanying fiber and nutrients.

Here are some key points and guidelines often associated with a no sugar diet:

- *Avoid added sugars:* This includes table sugar, high-fructose corn syrup, honey, maple syrup, agave nectar, and other sweeteners added to foods and beverages.

- *Read labels:* Pay attention to food labels and ingredient lists to identify hidden sources of sugar. Keep in mind that sugar can be listed under various names, such as sucrose, dextrose, fructose, and maltose.

- *Limit processed foods:* Many processed and packaged foods contain added sugars, so it's advisable to minimize consumption of items like candy, soda, baked goods, sugary cereals, and sweetened beverages.

- *Choose whole foods:* Focus on consuming whole, unprocessed foods such as fruits, vegetables, lean proteins, whole grains, and healthy fats. These foods tend to be lower in added sugars and higher in essential nutrients.

- *Be cautious of artificial sweeteners:* While artificial sweeteners may offer lower or zero-calorie alternatives, they are intensely sweet and can perpetuate cravings for sugary foods. It's best to minimize their use or opt for natural sweeteners like stevia or monk fruit in moderation.

- *Stay hydrated:* Drink plenty of water throughout the day to help maintain hydration and reduce the desire for sugary beverages.

- **_Plan meals and snacks:_** Prepare meals and snacks ahead of time to ensure you have healthy options available and avoid relying on processed or sugary foods when hunger strikes.

- **_Seek support:_** If you find it challenging to transition to a no sugar diet, consider seeking support from a nutritionist, joining a support group, or engaging with online communities that share similar goals.

It's important to consult with a healthcare professional or registered dietitian before making significant changes to your diet, especially if you have any underlying health conditions or dietary restrictions. They can provide personalized guidance and ensure you're meeting your nutritional needs while following a no sugar diet

Chapter 10: Real food is real Medicine

Here are 20 herbs and 20 vegetables known for their potential health benefits and ability to support wellness. It's important to note that individual needs and responses to these herbs and vegetables may vary. Always consult with a healthcare professional before incorporating new herbs or making significant changes to your diet.

Herbs

- **Turmeric:** Known for its anti-inflammatory properties.
- **Ginger:** Often used for digestive health and nausea relief.
- **Garlic:** Has potential antimicrobial and immune-boosting properties.
- **Cinnamon:** May help regulate blood sugar levels and improve insulin sensitivity.
- **Peppermint:** Used for digestive issues and soothing effects.

- **Chamomile:** Known for its calming and relaxation properties.
- **Echinacea:** Often used to support the immune system.
- **Ashwagandha:** An adaptogenic herb believed to support stress management.
- **Holy Basil (Tulsi):** Known for its antioxidant and stress-reducing properties.
- **Rosemary:** Contains compounds that may support cognitive function and memory.
- **Sage:** May have antioxidant and anti-inflammatory properties.
- **Oregano:** Known for its antimicrobial and antifungal properties.
- **Dandelion:** Often used to support liver health and digestion.
- **Milk Thistle:** Believed to have liver-protective properties.
- **Ginseng:** Known as an adaptogenic herb, often used for energy and stress management.
- **Licorice Root:** May help soothe digestive issues and support adrenal health.
- **Stinging Nettle:** Known for its potential anti-inflammatory and allergy-fighting effects.
- **Lavender:** Often used for relaxation and sleep support.
- **Lemon Balm:** Known for its calming and mood-enhancing effects.
- **Passionflower:** May help promote relaxation and reduce anxiety.

Vegetables:

- **Spinach:** Rich in vitamins, minerals, and antioxidants.
- **Broccoli:** Contains various nutrients and potential anti-cancer properties.
- **Kale:** Packed with vitamins, minerals, and antioxidants.
- **Bell peppers:** High in vitamin C and other beneficial compounds.

- **Carrots:** Rich in beta-carotene, known for promoting eye health.
- **Tomatoes:** Contain lycopene, a powerful antioxidant.
- **Cabbage:** May have anti-inflammatory and digestive health benefits.
- **Brussels sprouts:** Rich in fiber, vitamins, and minerals.
- **Sweet potatoes:** High in fiber, vitamins, and antioxidants.
- **Cauliflower:** Contains nutrients and potential anti-cancer properties.
- **Beets:** Known for their potential blood pressure-lowering effects and antioxidant properties.
- **Asparagus:** High in fiber and various vitamins and minerals.
- **Garlic:** May offer immune-boosting and heart health benefits.
- **Onions:** Contain compounds with potential anti-inflammatory and antimicrobial properties.
- **Green peas:** Packed with fiber, vitamins, and plant-based protein.
- **Zucchini:** Low in calories and a good source of vitamins and minerals.
- **Cucumbers:** Hydrating and low in calories, with potential anti-inflammatory effects.
- **Avocado:** Rich in healthy fats and various vitamins and minerals.
- **Radishes:** Provide fiber, vitamins, and potential anti-inflammatory benefits.
- **Mushrooms:** Contain beneficial compounds that may support immune health and offer antioxidant properties.

Meals:

1. **Nyoyo:** A dish made with cowpeas leaves cooked in a flavorful sauce with onions, tomatoes, and spices.
2. **Kunde na Ugali:** Cowpeas leaves cooked with onions, tomatoes, and spices, served with ugali.

3. **Kanzira:** A dish made with pumpkin leaves cooked with groundnuts (peanuts) and spices.
4. **Sukumawiki na Ndengu:** Collard greens cooked with pigeon peas, onions, tomatoes, and spices.
5. **Mchicha:** A dish made with amaranth leaves cooked with onions, tomatoes, and spices.
6. **Sukumawiki na Maharagwe:** Collard greens cooked with kidney beans, onions, tomatoes, and spices.
7. **Bhajia za Kunde:** Fried cowpeas fritters made with ground cowpeas, onions, and spices.
8. **Mrenda:** A dish made with moringa leaves cooked with onions, tomatoes, and spices.
9. **Saget na Maharagwe:** Jute mallow leaves cooked with kidney beans, onions, tomatoes, and spices.
10. **Pounded Yam with Vegetable Soup:** Yam pounded to a smooth consistency served with a flavorful vegetable soup made with assorted vegetables.
11. **Fried Sukumawiki:** Collard greens stir-fried with onions, tomatoes, garlic, and spices.
12. **Nduma na Nyanya:** Arrowroot tubers cooked with tomatoes, onions, and spices.
13. **Sukuma Bhajia na Brown Chapati:** A combination of mixed greens (kale, spinach, collard greens) cooked with onions, tomatoes, and spices, served with chapati.
14. **Mchicha na Uji:** Amaranth leaves cooked with millet or maize flour to make a thick porridge-like dish.
15. **Terere na Wali:** Amaranth leaves cooked with rice, onions, tomatoes, and spices.
16. **Sukuma Wiki na Njahi:** Collard greens cooked with black beans, onions, tomatoes, and spices.
17. **Dengu na Mchicha:** Pigeon peas cooked with amaranth leaves, onions, tomatoes, and spices.
18. **Biringanya za Nazi:** Eggplant cooked in a coconut sauce with onions, tomatoes, and spices.

19. **Majani ya Mchicha:** Tender amaranth leaves cooked with onions, tomatoes, and spices.
20. **Mchicha na Mboga:** Amaranth leaves cooked with mixed vegetables like carrots, green beans, and potatoes, flavored with onions, tomatoes, and spices.
21. **Majani ya Njugu:** Groundnut leaves cooked with onions, tomatoes, and spices.
22. **Maharagwe ya Nazi:** Kidney beans cooked in a creamy coconut sauce with onions, tomatoes, and spices.
23. **Kunde na Matoke:** Cowpeas leaves cooked with green bananas, onions, tomatoes, and spices.
24. **Kachumbari ya Nazi:** A coconut-based salad made with diced tomatoes, onions, cilantro, and coconut flakes.
25. **Sukuma Wiki na Kachumbari:** Collard greens served with a side of fresh tomato and onion salad.
26. **Kunde na Mrenda:** Cowpeas leaves cooked with moringa leaves, onions, tomatoes, and spices.
27. **Kunde na Irio:** Cowpeas leaves cooked with mashed peas, maize, and potatoes, flavored with onions and spices.
28. **Saget na Matoke:** Jute mallow leaves cooked with green bananas, onions, tomatoes, and spices.
29. **Kienyeji Mboga:** Traditional mixed vegetables like saget, terere, kunde, and mrenda cooked with onions, tomatoes, and spices.
30. **Mchicha na Ugali:** Amaranth leaves served with ugali.
31. **Pounded Cassava Leaves:** Cassava leaves pounded and cooked with onions, tomatoes, and spices.
32. **Dengu na Kachumbari:** Pigeon peas served with a side of fresh tomato and onion salad.
33. **Mboga za Nazi:** Mixed vegetables cooked in a coconut milk-based sauce with onions, tomatoes, and spices.
34. **Maboga ya Kienyeji:** Indigenous traditional greens like saget, terere, mrenda, and kunde cooked with onions, tomatoes, and spices.

35. **Viazi Karai:** Spiced and fried potato slices served with a tangy tomato and chili dip.
36. **Sukumawiki na Samaki:** Collard greens cooked with fish, onions, tomatoes, and spices.
37. **Sukuma Wiki na Viazi:** Collard greens cooked with potatoes, onions, tomatoes, and spices.
38. **Mrenda na Samaki:** Moringa leaves cooked with fish, onions, tomatoes, and spices.
39. Sukumawiki na Kachumbari: Collard greens served with a side of fresh tomato and onion salad.
40. **Mchicha na Kunde:** Amaranth leaves cooked with cowpeas, onions, tomatoes, and spices.

Incorporating a variety of herbs and vegetables into a balanced diet can provide a range of nutrients and potential health benefits. Remember to consume them as part of a well-rounded diet and consult with a healthcare professional for personalized guidance

Fruits:

1. *Avocado:* Rich in healthy fats, fiber, vitamins, and minerals. Avocados are associated with heart health and may help lower cholesterol levels.

2. *Mango:* Packed with vitamins A and C, mangoes are known for their antioxidant properties and may support immune function and eye health.

3. *Papaya:* Contains a digestive enzyme called papain and is a good source of vitamin C and folate. Papaya may aid digestion and promote healthy skin.

4. *Pineapple:* Contains bromelain, an enzyme that aids digestion, and is a good source of vitamin C. Pineapple may have anti-inflammatory properties.

5. **_Watermelon:_** Hydrating and low in calories, watermelon is rich in lycopene, an antioxidant that may help reduce the risk of certain cancers.

6. **_Passion Fruit:_** Packed with vitamins A and C, passion fruit is known for its antioxidant properties and may support immune health.

7. **_Banana:_** High in potassium, fiber, and vitamin C, bananas are known for their heart-healthy properties and may help regulate blood pressure.

8. **_Guava:_** Rich in vitamin C, fiber, and antioxidants, guava may support immune function and digestive health.

9. **_Berries (e.g strawberries, raspberries, blackberries):_** Loaded with antioxidants, vitamins, and fiber, berries are associated with various health benefits, including reduced inflammation and improved heart health.

10. **_Oranges:_** High in vitamin C and fiber, oranges are known for their immune-boosting properties and may help reduce the risk of chronic diseases.

11. **_Lemons:_** Rich in vitamin C and antioxidants, lemons may aid digestion and support immune function.

12. **_Pawpaw (Papaya):_** Contains digestive enzymes and is rich in vitamins A and C, which promote healthy digestion and immune health.

It's important to note that while these fruits offer potential health benefits, a balanced and varied diet, along with a healthy lifestyle, is crucial for overall well-being and the prevention of chronic diseases.

Chapter11: Nurturing a Healthy Lifestyle

Nurturing a healthy lifestyle is a lifelong commitment to taking care of your physical, mental, and emotional well-being. It involves making conscious choices that promote overall health and vitality. Here are some key aspects to consider when nurturing a healthy lifestyle:

Balanced Diet: Focus on consuming a balanced and nutritious diet that includes a variety of whole foods such as fruits, vegetables, whole grains, lean proteins, and healthy fats. Avoid excessive consumption of processed foods, sugary snacks, and drinks. Practice portion control and mindful eating.

Regular Physical Activity: Engage in regular physical activity that suits your fitness level and preferences. Aim for a combination of cardiovascular exercises, strength training, and flexibility exercises. Find activities that you enjoy, such as walking, jogging, swimming, cycling, dancing, or playing sports. Remember to consult with a healthcare professional before starting any new exercise program.

Adequate Sleep: Prioritize getting enough quality sleep each night. Establish a consistent sleep schedule, create a sleep-friendly environment, and practice relaxation techniques to promote restful sleep. Aim for 7-9 hours of sleep for adults.

Stress Management: Adopt effective stress management techniques to minimize the negative impact of stress on your health. Explore stress-reducing activities such as meditation, deep breathing exercises, yoga, mindfulness practices, journaling, or engaging in hobbies that bring you joy.

Hydration: Stay adequately hydrated by drinking plenty of water throughout the day. Water helps maintain optimal bodily functions, supports digestion, and aids in the elimination of toxins.

Emotional Well-being: Take care of your mental and emotional health. Seek support from loved ones, cultivate healthy relationships, practice self-care, engage in activities that bring you happiness, and consider professional help if needed.

Avoid Alcohol and Tobacco Use: If you consume alcohol, do so in moderation. Avoid tobacco and limit exposure to secondhand smoke. These substances can have detrimental effects on your health.

Regular Health Check-ups: Schedule routine check-ups and screenings with your healthcare provider to monitor your health and detect any potential issues early on. Address any concerns or symptoms promptly.

Positive Mindset: Cultivate a positive mindset and practice self-compassion. Focus on gratitude, positive affirmations, and maintaining a healthy perspective on life's challenges.

Social Connection: Nurture your social connections and engage in activities that foster a sense of belonging and community. Spend time with loved ones, join social or hobby groups, and support others in their wellness journeys.

Conclusion

In conclusion, the excessive consumption of sugar has become a global health concern with far-reaching consequences. Obesity and metabolic syndrome, both closely linked to sugar intake, have become widespread epidemics, affecting millions of individuals worldwide. The impact of excessive sugar consumption on our health cannot be ignored.

However, there is hope for a sweet and balanced future. By raising awareness about the dangers of sugar and its connection to chronic diseases, we can empower individuals to make informed choices and take control of their health. It is crucial to promote healthier eating habits, emphasizing the importance of real, nutrient-dense foods in our diets.

Education and advocacy play vital roles in addressing this global health concern. Governments, healthcare professionals, and communities must work together to implement policies and initiatives that promote healthy eating habits and reduce sugar consumption. Access to affordable and nutritious food options must be prioritized, ensuring that everyone has the opportunity to make healthier choices.

Additionally, individuals can take proactive steps in their own lives to reduce sugar intake. This includes reading food labels, avoiding processed and sugary foods, and opting for natural alternatives. By adopting a balanced and mindful approach to nutrition, we can reclaim our health and prevent the onset of chronic diseases.

A sweet and balanced future lies ahead, where individuals are empowered to make healthier choices and embrace a lifestyle that nurtures their well-being. By prioritizing real, whole foods and reducing our reliance on processed sugars, we can pave the way for a healthier and happier society. Let us embark on this journey together, promoting a future where sugar is consumed in moderation, and chronic diseases are significantly reduced. Together, we can create a future where health and well-being flourish.

Reference

Scientific research has provided evidence supporting the harmful effects of excessive consumption of processed sugar on health. Here are some key findings from scientific studies:

Obesity and Weight Gain: Numerous studies have linked high sugar intake to weight gain and obesity. Excessive sugar consumption contributes to increased calorie intake, reduced satiety (feeling full), and a higher risk of developing metabolic disorders.

- Malik, V. S., Popkin, B. M., Bray, G. A., Després, J. P., Willett, W. C., & Hu, F. B. (2010). Sugar-sweetened beverages, obesity, type 2 diabetes mellitus, and cardiovascular disease risk. Circulation, 121(11), 1356-1364.

- Malik, V. S., Schulze, M. B., & Hu, F. B. (2006). Intake of sugar-sweetened beverages and risk of type 2 diabetes: A systematic review. Diabetes Care, 29(5), 1343-1348.
- Yang, Q., Zhang, Z., Gregg, E. W., Flanders, W. D., Merritt, R., & Hu, F. B. (2014). Added sugar intake and cardiovascular diseases mortality among US adults. JAMA Internal Medicine, 174(4), 516-524.
- Moynihan, P., & Petersen, P. E. (2004). Diet, nutrition and the prevention of dental diseases. Public Health Nutrition, 7(1A), 201-226.

Non-Alcoholic Fatty Liver Disease (NAFLD): Excessive sugar consumption, especially in the form of fructose, has been associated with an increased risk of developing NAFLD. Consuming high amounts of fructose can lead to fat accumulation in the liver and insulin resistance.

- Basaranoglu, M., Basaranoglu, G., & Bugianesi, E. (2013). Carbohydrate intake and nonalcoholic fatty liver disease: Fructose as a weapon of mass destruction. Hepatobiliary Surgery and Nutrition, 2(2), 109-116.

These studies and many others provide evidence of the detrimental effects of excessive consumption of processed sugar on health. Reducing added sugar intake and focusing on a balanced, whole-foods diet can contribute to improved health outcomes.